CW00520061

The Complete Healthy Instant Pot Cookbook

The Ultimate Complete Healthy Instant Pot Cookbook with Delicious Whole-Food Recipes for your Pressure Cooker, for Eat Healthy Light Meals

Brian Smith

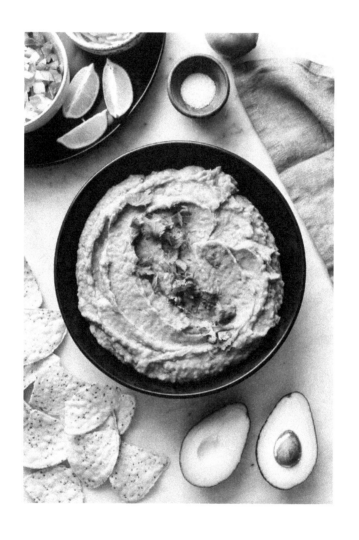

Table of Contents

consent from the Publisher. All additional right reserved.The information in the following pages is broadly considered a truthful and accurate account of facts and as such, any inattention, use, or misuse of the information in question by the reader will render any resulting actions solely under their purview. There are no scenarios in which the publisher or the original author of this work can be in any fashion deemed liable for any hardship or damages that may befall them after undertaking information described herein. Additionally, the information in the following pages is intended only for informational purposes and should thus be thought of as universal. As befitting its nature, it is presented without assurance regarding its prolonged validity or interim quality. Trademarks that are mentioned are done without written consent and can in no way be considered an endorsement from the trademark holder.

Introduction

Instant pot is a pressure cooker, also stir-fry, stew, and cook rice, cook vegetables and chicken. It's an all-in-one device, so you can season chicken and cook it in the same pan, for example. In most cases, instant pot meals can be served in less than an hour.

Cooking less time is due to the pressure cooking function that captures the steam generated by the liquid cooking environment (including liquids released from meat and vegetables), boosts the pressure and pushes the steam back.

But don't confuse with traditional pressure cookers. The instant pot, unlike the pressure cooker used by grandparents, eliminates the risk of safety with a lid that locks and remains locked until pressure is released.

Even when cooking time is over in the instant pot, you need to take an additional step-to release the pressure.

There are two ways to relieve pressure. Due to the natural pressure release, the lid valve remains in the sealing position and the pressure will naturally dissipate over time. This process takes 20 minutes to over an hour, depending on what is cooked. Low fluidity foods (such as chicken wings) take less time than high fluidity foods such as soups and marinades.

Another option is manual pressure release (also called quick release). Now you need to carefully move the valve to the ventilation position and see that the steam rises slowly and the pressure is released. This Directions is much faster, but foods with high liquid content, such as soups, take about 15 minutes to manually relieve pressure.

Which option should I use? Take into account that even if natural pressure is released, the instant pot is still under pressure. This means that the food will continue to cook while the instant pot is in sealed mode. Manual pressure relief is useful when the dishes are well cooked and need to be stopped as soon as possible.

If the goal is to prepare meals quickly, set the cooking time for dishes that are being cooked in an instant pop and release the pressure manually after the time has passed.

Instant pots (called "Instapot" by many) are one of our favorite cookware because they can handle such a wide range of foods almost easily. Instant pots range from those that work on the basics of pressure cooking to those that can be sterilized using Suicide video or some models can be controlled via Wi-Fi.

In addition, if you want to expand the range of kitchenware, the Instant Pot brand has released an air fryer that can be used to make rotisserie chicken and homemade beef jerky. There is also an independent accumulator device that can be used in instant pots to make fish, steaks and more.

The current icon instant pot works like a pressure cooker and uses heat and steam to quickly cook food. Everything from perfect carnitas to boiled eggs was cooked, but not all ingredients and DIRECTIONSs work. Here are few foods that should not be cooked in classic instant pots.

Instant pots are not pressure fryer and are not designed to handle the high temperatures required to heat cooking oils like crispy fried chicken. Of course, the instant pot is great for dishes like Carnitas, but after removing the meat from the instant pot, to get the final crispness in the meat, transfer it to a frying pan for a few minutes or to an oven top and hot Crispy in the oven.

As with slow cookers, dairy products such as cheese, milk, and sour cream will pack into instant pots using pressure cooking settings or slow cooking settings. Do not add these ingredients after the dish are cooked or create a recipe in Instapot.

There are two exceptions. One is when making yogurt. This is merely possible if you are using an instant pot recipe. The other is only when making cheesecake and following an instant pot recipe.

Although you can technically cook pasta in an instant pot, gummy may appear and cooking may be uneven. To be honest, unless you have a choice, cooking pasta in a stove pot is just as fast and easy and consistently gives you better cooked pasta.

Instead of baking the cake in an instant pot, steam it. The cake is moist-it works for things like bread pudding-but there is no good skin on the cake or on the crunchy edge everyone fights with a baked brownie. However, let's say your desire is to build a close-up or a simple dessert with your family; you can get a damp sponge in about 30 minutes, except during the DIRECTIONS time.

Canning, a technique for cooking and sealing food in a jar, is often done in a pressure cooker. Therefore, it is recommended to create a batch of jam, pickles or jelly in Instapot. Please do not.

With an instant pot, you can't monitor the temperature of what you can, like a normal pressure cooker. In canning, it is important to cook and seal the dishes correctly. Incorrect cooking and sealing can lead to the growth of bacteria that can cause food poisoning.

If you want to avoid canning in an instant pot, some newer models, such as Duo Plus, have a sterilization setting that can clean kitchen items such as baby bottles, bottles and cookware.

Instant Pot Pressure Cooker Safety Tips

Instant Pot is a very safe pressure cooker consisting of various safety mechanisms. do not worry. It will not explode immediately. Most accidents are caused by user errors and can be easily avoided. To further minimize the possibility of an accident, we have compiled a list of safety tips.

1 Don't leave it alone

It is not recommended to leave home while cooking an instant pot. If you have to leave it alone, make sure it is under pressure and no steam is coming out.

2 Do not use KFC in instant pot

Do not fry in an instant pot or other pressure cooker.

KFC uses a commercial pressure fryer specially made to fry chicken (the latest one that operates at 5 PSI). Instant pots (10.5-11.6 PSI) are specially made to make our lives easier.

3 water intake!

Instant pots require a minimum of 1 1/2 cup liquid (Instant Pot Official Number) 1 cup liquid to reach and maintain pressure.

The liquid can be a combination of gravy, vinegar, water, chicken etc.

4 half full or half empty

The max line printed on the inner pot of the instant pot is not for pressure cooking.

For pressure cooking: up to 2/3 full

Food for pressure cooking that expands during cooking (grains, beans, dried vegetables, etc.): up to 1/2

5 Not a facial steamer

Deep cleaning is not performed even if the pressure cooker steam is used once.

When opening, always tilt the lid away from you. Wear waterproof and heat-resistant silicone gloves especially when performing quick release.

6 never use power

In situations of zero, you should try to force open the lid of the instant pot pressure cooker, unless you want to prevent a light saber from hitting your face.

7 Wash Up & Checkout

If you want to be secured, wash the lid after each use and clean the anti-block shield and inner pot. Make sure that the gasket (silicon seal ring) is in good shape and that there is no food residue in the anti-block shield before use.

Usually silicone seal rings should be replaced every 18-24 months. It is always advisable to keep extra things.

Do not purchase a sealing ring from a third party because it is an integral part of the safety features of the instant ring.

Using sealing rings that have not been tested with instant pot products can create serious safety concerns."

Before use, make sure that the sealing ring is securely fixed to the sealing ring rack and the anti-block shield is properly attached to the vapor discharge pipe.

A properly fitted sealing ring can be moved clockwise or counterclockwise in the sealing ring rack with little force.

With instant pots, the whole family can cook meals in less than 30 minutes. Cooked dishes such as rice, chicken, beef stew, sauce, yakitori can be cooked for 30-60 minutes from the beginning to the end. And yes, you can bake bread in an instant pot.

Old and ketogenic diet fans love instant pots for their ability to `` roast '' meat in such a short time, but vegetarians and vegans that can quickly cook dishes such as pumpkin soup, baked potatoes and marinated potato chilis, also highly appreciated oatmeal cream and macaroni and cheese.

Even dried beans, which usually require overnight cooking, can be prepared in 30 minutes to make spicy hummus.

Breakfast

Acorn Squash

Preparation time: 15 minutes

Cooking time: 20 minutes

Servings: 4

Ingredients:

1 acorn squash

3 tbsp. Butter (melted

2 tsp. Brown sugar

1/2 tsp. Kosher salt

Black pepper to taste

Optional toppings: melted butter, roasted nuts (chopped), pomegranate seeds

Directions:

Cleanse squash and trim ends. Cut in half and core to remove seeds. Cut into about half an inch thick.

Combine in a bowl brown sugar, melted butter. Season with salt and pepper.

Add in the acorn squash and toss to coat.

Place coated squash into the air fryer basket and attach the air fryer lid to the instant pot. Set to air fry at 375 degrees Fahrenheit for 15-20 minutes or until tender, flipping after 10 minutes of cooking.

Once done, serve in a platter drizzled with melted butter, pomegranate seeds, and chopped nuts.

Taste for seasoning and adjust flavor if needed.

Nutrition:

Calories – 152 Kcal;

Fat – 7.73;

Carbohydrates – 27.74 G;

Protein –2.63 G;

Sugar –12.45 G;

Fiber – 4.6 G;

Sodium – 352 Mg

Instant Pot Air-Fried Avocado

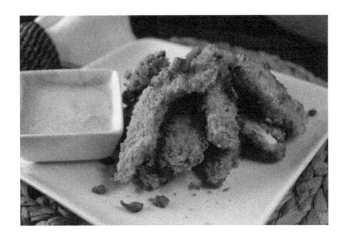

Preparation time: 10 minutes

Cooking time: 10 minutes

Servings: 2

Ingredients:

1/2 cup all-purpose flour

2 avocados

2 large eggs

2 tbsp. Canola mayonnaise

1 tbsp. Apple cider vinegar

1 tbsp. Sriracha chili sauce

1 1/2 tsp. Black pepper

1/4 tsp. Kosher salt

1/2 cup panko breadcrumbs

1/4 cup no-salt-added ketchup

1 tbsp. Water

Cooking spray

Directions:

Cut avocado into 4 wedges each. Prepare 3
shallow dishes.

In the first shallow dish, combine avocado wedges
with flour and pepper.

In another dish, lightly beat eggs

Place breadcrumbs in the third dish

First, dredge avocado wedges in the flour mixture,
one after the other. After coating with flour, shake
lightly to remove excess flour and dip the avocado
to the egg mixture, likewise shaking lightly to drip
off excess liquid. Finally, dip each wedge to the
breadcrumbs coating them evenly on all sides and
spray with cooking oil.

Arrange avocado wedged in the instant pot duo air fryer basket, place it inside the pot, and cover it with the air fryer lid. Set to 400 degrees F until wedges turn golden brown, turning them over halfway through cooking. Remove avocado wedges from the fryer and sprinkle it with salt. Meanwhile, while waiting for the avocado wedges to get cooked, mix mayonnaise, ketchup, apple cider vinegar, and sriracha sauce in a small bowl. Serve the prepared sauce with the avocado wedges while still warm.

Nutrition:

Calories – 274 Kcal; Fat – 18g; Carbohydrates – 23g; Protein –5g;Sugar –5g; Fiber – 7g; Sodium – 306mg

Mediterranean Veggies In Instant Pot Air Fryer

Preparation time: 5 minutes

Cooking time: 20 minutes

Servings: 4

Ingredients:

1 1 large courgetti

50 g cherry tomatoes

1 green pepper

1 medium carrot

1 large parsnip

1 tsp. Mixed herbs

2 tbsp. Honey

Tbsp. Olive oil

2 tsp. Garlic puree

1 tsp. Mustard

Salt and pepper to taste

Directions:

Slice up the courgetti and the green pepper.

Peel and dice the carrots and the parsnips

Add them all altogether in the air fryer basket of the instant pot duo along with raw cherry tomatoes. Drizzle with three tablespoons of olive oil.

Place the air fryer in the pot and air fry for 15 minutes at 356 degrees Fahrenheit using instant pot air fryer crisp air fryer. Dash with more salt if needed and serve.

Nutrition:

Calories – 281 Kcal;

Fat – 21g;

Carbohydrates – 21g;

Protein –2g;

Sugar –13g;

Fiber – 3g;

Sodium – 36mg

Rosemary air-fried potatoes

Preparation time: 10 minutes

Cooking time: 15 minutes

Servings: 4

Ingredients:

3 tbsp. Vegetable oil

4 yellow baby potatoes (quartered

2 tsp. Dried rosemary minced

1 tbsp. Minced garlic

1 tsp. Ground black pepper

1/4 cup chopped parsley

1 tbsp. Fresh lime or lemon juice

1 tsp. Salt

Directions:

Add potatoes, garlic, rosemary, pepper, and salt in a large bowl. Mix thoroughly.

Arrange seasoned potatoes in the air fryer basket and place it inside the instant pot duo. Cover with the air fryer lid and air fry at 400 degrees Fahrenheit for about 15 minutes.

Check to see if tomatoes are cooked through since it depends on the size of potatoes.

Once cooked, take it out of the air fryer and place in a platter.

Sprinkle with lemon juice and parsley.

Serve warm.

Nutrition:

Calories – 201 Kcal;

Fat – 10.71g;

Carbohydrates – 22.71g;

Protein –3.34g;

Sugar –1.32g;

Fiber – 3.5g;

Broccoli and Cauliflower Medley

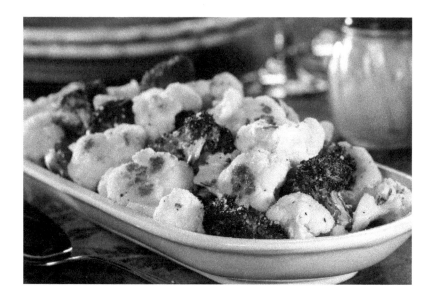

Preparation Time: 10 minutes

Cooking Time: 10 minutes

Serving: 2

Ingredients:

1/2 lb. broccoli fresh

1/2 lb. cauliflower fresh

1 tablespoon olive oil

1/4 teaspoon black pepper

1/4 teaspoon salt

1/4 teaspoon garlic salt

1/3 cup water

Directions:

Toss the vegetable with seasonings and olive oil in a bowl.

Pour 1/3 cup water into the Instant Pot duo base.

Place the Air fry basket inside and spread the vegetables in it.

Put on the Air Fryer lid and seal it.

Hit the "Roast Button" and select 10 minutes of cooking time, then press "Start."

Once the Instant Pot Duo beeps, remove its lid.

Serve.

Nutrition:

Calories 90

Total Fat 7g

Sodium 324mg

Total Carbohydrate 7.4g

Dietary Fiber 3.1g

Total Sugars 2.8g

Protein 3.1g

Roasted Squash Mix

Preparation Time: 10 minutes

Cooking Time: 40 minutes

Servings: 2

Ingredients:

3 potatoes, cubed

1 red onion, quartered

1 butternut squash, cubed

1 sweet potato, peeled and cubed

1 tablespoon fresh thyme, chopped

2 tablespoons fresh rosemary, chopped

2 red bell peppers, seeded and diced

1/4 cup olive oil

2 tablespoons balsamic vinegar

Salt and freshly ground black pepper

Directions:

Whisk rosemary with thyme, vinegar, olive oil, black pepper, and salt in a bowl.

Toss in onion, bell peppers, squash, potatoes, and sweet potato.

Add the vegetables to the Instant Pot Duo.

Put on the Air Fryer lid and seal it.

Hit the "Roast Button" and select 40 minutes of cooking time, then press "Start."

Toss the roasting vegetables every 10 minutes.

Once the Instant Pot Duo beeps, remove its lid.

Serve.

Nutrition:

Calories 570

Total Fat 26.7g

Saturated Fat 4g

Sodium 58mg

Total Carbohydrate 82.8g

Dietary Fiber 11.5g

Total Sugars 15.4g

Protein 9.2g

Zucchini Satay

Preparation Time: 10 minutes

Cooking Time: 10 minutes

Servings: 2

Ingredients:

2 zucchinis, sliced

2 yellow squash, sliced

1 container mushrooms, halved

1/2 cup olive oil

1/2 onion sliced

3/4 teaspoon Italian seasoning

1/2 teaspoon garlic salt

1/4 teaspoon seasoned salt

Directions:

Toss zucchini, squash, onion, and mushrooms in a large bowl.

Whisk olive oil, with Italian seasoning, salt, and garlic salt in a small bowl.

Pour this olive oil mixture into the vegetables then toss well.

Spread the seasoned veggies in the Air Fryer Basket.

Set the Air Fryer Basket in the Instant Pot Duo.

Put on the Air Fryer lid and seal it.

Hit the "Air fry Button" and select 10 minutes of cooking time, then press "Start."

Once the Instant Pot Duo beeps, remove its lid. Serve.

Nutrition:

Calories 492

Total Fat 51.4g

Saturated Fat 7.4g

Cholesterol 1mg

Sodium 22mg

Total Carbohydrate 11.8g

Dietary Fiber 4.2g

Total Sugars 5.5g

Protein 4.7g

Cauliflower Cheese Pasta

Preparation Time: 10 minutes

Cooking Time: 27 minutes

Servings: 4

Ingredients:

9 oz. shell pasta, cooked and drained

3.5 oz. unsalted butter

2 bay leaves

1 onion, chopped

3 garlic cloves, crushed

1/2 bunch sage, chopped

1 tbsp plain flour

3 3/4 cups cream

7 oz. smoked cheese, coarsely grated

1 1/4 cups parmesan, grated

1 large cauliflower, blanched, cut into wedges

1/4 teaspoon nutmeg, grated

Directions:

Place a frypan over medium-high heat and add butter.

Melt it and add garlic, onion, and bay leave then sauté for 5 minutes.

Discard the bay leaves, then stir in flour and sage. Stir cook for 2 minutes.

Slowly add cream, cheese, pasta, and parmesan, then add crumbled cauliflower.

Stir in nutmeg and seasoning, then transfer to the Instant Pot Duo.

Put on the Air Fryer lid and seal it.

Hit the "Bake Button" and select 20 minutes of cooking time, then press "Start."

Once the Instant Pot Duo beeps, remove its lid. Serve.

Nutrition:

Calories 427

Total Fat 23.8g

Saturated Fat 14.4g

Cholesterol 106mg

Sodium 263mg

Total Carbohydrate 43.1g

Dietary Fiber 2.5g

Total Sugars 2.9g, Protein 12.1g

Pumpkin Baked Gnocchi

Preparation Time: 10 minutes

Cooking Time: 46 minutes

Servings: 6

Ingredients:

26 oz. potato gnocchi, cooked

1/3 cup olive oil

16 sage leaves

26 oz. pumpkin, cut into slices

2 egg yolks

2 ½ cup cream

1/2 teaspoon finely grated nutmeg

3/4 cup coarsely grated mozzarella

3.5 oz. blue cheese, crumbled

Roasted chopped hazelnuts, to serve

Directions:

Mix pumpkin with 1 tablespoon oil in a bowl.

Stir in egg yolks, cream, gnocchi, half of the sage, half of the blue cheese, nutmeg, cream, and mozzarella.

Spread this mixture in the Instant Pot Duo insert.

Top the casserole with remaining cheese.

Put on the Air Fryer lid and seal it.

Hit the "Bake Button" and select 45 minutes of cooking time, then press "Start."

Once the Instant Pot Duo beeps, remove its lid.

Heat ¼ cup in a frying pan and add sage. Sauté for 1 minute.

Transfer the fried sage to a plate lined with a paper towel.

Add this fried sage, and nuts to the casserole.

Garnish with sage oil.

Serve.

Nutrition:

Calories 537

Total Fat 30.8g

Saturated Fat 13g

Cholesterol 122mg

Sodium 560mg

Total Carbohydrate 50.1g

Dietary Fiber 0.8g

Total Sugars 0.9g

Protein 17.8g

Pumpkin Lasagna

Preparation Time: 10 minutes

Cooking Time: 60 minutes

Servings: 6

Ingredients:

28 oz. pumpkin, cut into slices

1 bunch sage, chopped

1/2 cup ghee, melted

1 leek, thinly sliced

4 garlic cloves, finely grated

3.5 oz. kale and cavolo Nero leaves shredded

270g semi-dried tomatoes, drained, chopped

17 0z. quark

2 eggs, lightly beaten

Directions:

Mix pumpkin slices with sage leaves, 2 teaspoon salt, 2 tablespoon ghee in a bowl.

Toss leek separately with 2 tablespoon ghee, garlic, and ½ teaspoon salt in another bowl.

Mix kale with 1 teaspoon salt, tomato, and cavolo Nero in a bowl.

Now beat eggs with quark and sage in a bowl.

Take a baking pan that can fit into the Instant Pot Duo.

Add 1/3 of the leek mixture at the base of the baking pan.

Top this mixture with a layer of pumpkin slices.

Add 1/3 of quark mixture on top then add 1/3 of kale mixture over it.

Top it with pumpkin slices and continue repeating the layer while ending at the pumpkin slice layer on top.

Place the baking pan in the Instant Pot duo.

Put on the Air Fryer lid and seal it.

Hit the "Bake Button" and select 60 minutes of cooking time, then press "Start."

Once the Instant Pot Duo beeps, remove its lid.

Serve.

Nutrition:

Calories 491

Total Fat 29.9g

Saturated Fat 16.9g

Total Carbohydrate 52.1g, Protein 14.8g

Haloumi Baked Rusti

Preparation Time: 10 minutes

Cooking Time: 35 minutes

Servings: 4

Ingredients:

Olive oil, to brush

7 oz. sweet potato, coarsely grated

10 oz. potatoes, coarsely grated

10 oz. carrots, coarsely grated

9 oz. halloumi, coarsely grated

1/2 onion, coarsely grated

2 tbsp thyme leaves

2 eggs

1/3 cup plain flour

1/2 cup sour cream, to serve

Fennel Salad

2 celery stalks, thinly sliced

1 fennel, thinly sliced

1/2 cup olives, chopped

Juice of 1 lemon

1 lemon quarter, chopped

1 teaspoon toasted coriander seeds, ground

Directions:

Toss sweet potato, carrot, potato, onion, halloumi, thyme, flour, and eggs in a bowl.

Spread this mixture in the Instant Pot Duo insert.

Put on the Air Fryer lid and seal it.

Hit the "Bake Button" and select 35 minutes of cooking time, then press "Start."

Once the Instant Pot Duo beeps, remove its lid.

Prepare the salad by mixing its Ingredients: in a salad bowl.

Serve the sweet potato rosti with the prepared salad.

Nutrition:

Calories 462

Total Fat 21.1g

Total Carbohydrate 43.9g

Protein 23g

Celeriac Potato Gratin

Preparation Time: 10 minutes

Cooking Time: 63 minutes

Servings: 6

Ingredients:

2 cups cream

1 teaspoon caraway seeds, toasted

1 garlic clove, crushed

1 teaspoon fennel seeds, toasted

2 bay leaves

1/4 teaspoon ground cloves

Zest of 1/2 a lemon

2 teaspoon melted butter

1kg potatoes, peeled

1 cup celeriac, peeled and minced

6 slices prosciutto, torn

3/4 cup fresh ricotta

¼ cup fontina cheese, grated

Directions:

Add cream, garlic, caraway seeds, cloves, bay leaves, fennel, zest, and cloves to a saucepan.

Stir cook this mixture for 3 minutes then remove from the heat.

Thinly slices potato by passing through the mandolin and spread the potatoes in the insert of Instant Pot Duo.

Top the potato with celeriac, prepared white sauce, prosciutto, and ricotta.

Put on the Air Fryer lid and seal it.

Hit the "Bake Button" and select 60 minutes of cooking time, then press "Start."

Once the Instant Pot Duo beeps, remove its lid.

Serve.

Nutrition:

Calories 399

Total Fat 20.3g

Total Carbohydrate 23.6g

Protein 31.3g

Eggplant Pine Nut Roast

Preparation Time: 10 minutes

Cooking Time: 66 minutes

Servings: 6

Ingredients:

6 Japanese eggplants

2/3 cup olive oil

1 onion, finely chopped

4 garlic cloves, crushed

1 1/2 tbsp sundried tomato pesto

1 teaspoon smoked paprika

14 oz. can cherry tomatoes

1 teaspoon zaatar, plus extra to serve

2/3 cup vegetable stock

1/2 bunch mint, chopped

2 tbsp toasted pine nuts, roughly crushed

1/4 cup Greek yogurt

Juice of 1 lemon

Directions:

Add eggplants to the Air Fryer Basket and pour 2 tablespoon oil over them.

Set the Air Fryer Basket in the Instant Pot Duo.

Put on the Air Fryer lid and seal it.

Hit the "Bake Button" and select 30 minutes of cooking time, then press "Start."

Once the Instant Pot Duo beeps, remove its lid.

Meanwhile, prepare the sauce by sautéing onion with remaining oil in a pan.

After 4 minutes, add garlic to sauté for 2 minutes.

Add tomato, stock, zaatar, paprika and tomato pesto.

Cook this sauce for 10 minutes until it thickens.

Pour this sauce over the eggplant and continue baking it for another 20 minutes.

Mix yogurt with lemon juice, mint, and pine nuts.

Serve the baked eggplants with yogurt.

Nutrition:

Calories 413

Total Fat 25g

Total Carbohydrate 45g

Protein 9.2g

Roasted Veggie Casserole

Preparation Time: 10 minutes

Cooking Time: 50 minutes

Servings: 6

Ingredients:

½ head cauliflower, cut into chunks

1 sweet potato, peeled and cubed

2 red bell peppers, cubed

1 yellow onion, sliced

3 tablespoons olive oil

1 teaspoon ground cumin

Salt

Freshly ground black pepper

2 ¼ cups red salsa

½ cup chopped fresh cilantro

9 corn tortillas cut in half

1 can (15 oz.) black beans, drained

2 big handfuls (about 2 oz.) baby spinach leaves

2 cups Monterey Jack cheese, shredded

Directions:

Toss the vegetables with olive oil, salt, black pepper, and cumin in a large bowl.

Add these vegetables to the Air Fryer Basket and set it inside the Instant Pot Duo.

Put on the Air Fryer lid and seal it.

Hit the "Bake Button" and select 30 minutes of cooking time, then press "Start."

Once the Instant Pot Duo beeps, remove its lid.

Transfer the veggies to a baking pan and top it with salsa, tortilla, beans, spinach, and cheese.

Place this pan in the Instant Pot Duo.

Put on the Air Fryer lid and seal it.

Hit the "Bake Button" and select 20 minutes of cooking time, then press "Start."

Once the Instant Pot Duo beeps, remove its lid.

Serve.

Nutrition:

Calories 390

Total Fat 20.5g

Total Carbohydrate 38.7g

Protein 15.8g

Air Fryer Crispy Broccoli

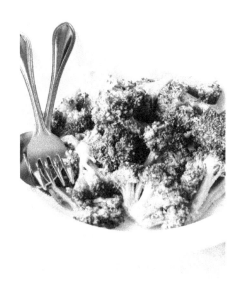

Preparation time: 5 minutes

Cooking time: 10 minutes

Servings: 4

Ingredients:

2 tbsp. Cooking oil

1 lb. Broccoli (cut into bite-size pieces

½ tsp. Garlic powder

Salt and pepper to taste

Fresh lemon wedges

Directions

Put the broccoli in a bowl and drizzle evenly with olive oil.

Season broccoli with garlic powder, salt, and pepper.

Put in instant pot air fryer crisp air fryer basket and cover with the air fryer lid.

Air fry 380degrees Fahrenheit for 12-15 minutes, flipping and shaking 3 times through cooking or cook until crispy.

Serve with lemon wedges.

Nutrition:

Calories – 104 Kcal;

Fat – 7.41g;

Carbohydrates – 5.42 G;

 Protein –3.93 G;

Healthy Coconut Yogurt

Preparation Time: 5 minutes

Cooking Time: 10 minutes

Servings: 6

Ingredients:

Coconut cream2 cans

Probiotic4 capsules

Directions:

First, pour the coconut cream into the cooker. Press the Yogurt button and when it comes to a boil, open the lid and watch the temperature. When the temperature reaches 120 F, open the capsules and add the powder to the instant pot. Stir to mix the powder with the cream.

Make sure to lock the lid and choose the yogurt button. Adjust the time to 15 hours. Leave. When finished, pour the yogurt into a bowl and transfer to your refrigerator for a day.

Nutrition:

Calories – 170,Protein – 5 g. Fat – 1.4 g. Carbs – 33 g.

Oatmeal with Caramelized Bananas

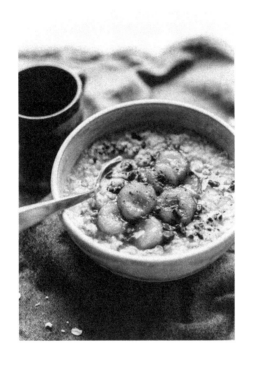

Preparation Time: 5 minutes

Cooking Time: 20 minutes

Servings: 4

Ingredients:

Oats1 cup

Milk1 cup

Water1.5 cups

Peanut butter1/3 cup

Bananas 2

Butter1 tbsp.

Directions:

Put the first three ingredients into the instant pot and close the lid. Manually set the time for 8 minutes at high pressure. Allow to cook.

Meanwhile, slice the banana and melt the butter. Turn off the cooker and naturally release the pressure. Add the butter and stir well.

Serve with topping of banana and chocolate chips.

Nutrition:

Calories – 330

Protein – 7 g.

Fat – 12 g.

Carbs – 51 g.

Easy Homemade Oats

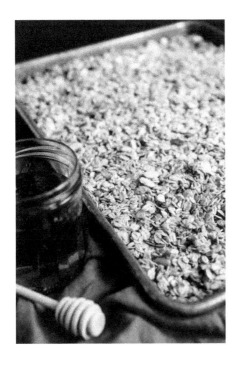

Preparation Time: 5 minutes

Cooking Time: 12 minutes

Servings: 4

Ingredients:

Steel cut oats1 cup

Brown sugar¼ cup

Butter2 tbsp.

Salt1 pinch

Water3 cups

Cranberries½ cup

Slivered almonds½ cup

Directions:

Take your instant pot and add the butter, brown sugar, salt, water, and oats. Stir and close the lid. Set the cooking time to 12 minutes.

Release the pressure and stir to desired consistency.

Serve with topping of cranberries and almonds.

Nutrition:

Calories – 140

Protein – 4 g.

Fat – 2.5 g.

Carbs – 26 g.

Healthy Instant Oats with Fruit

Preparation Time: 5 minutes

Cooking Time: 15 minutes

Servings: 2

Ingredients:

Steel cut oats1 cup

Water1. 5 cups.

Butter2 tbsp.

Orange juice1 cup

Cranberries1 tbsp.

Raisins1 tbsp.

Dried apricots1 tbsp.

Maple syrup2 tbsp.

Cinnamon¼ tsp.

Pecans2 tbsp.

Salt to taste

Directions:

Add the all ingredients in the instant pot and stir to combine well. Make sure to lock the lid and manually set the time for 10 minutes.

Open the cover, stir everything and transfer to the serving cups.

Nutrition:

Calories – 98

Protein – 1.3 g.

Fat – 4 g.

Carbs – 14 g.

Energetic Boiled Egg

Preparation Time: 5 minutes

Cooking Time: 15 minutes

Servings: 2

Ingredients:

Egg2

Water1 cup

Directions:

Take your instant pot and add the rack comes with it. Pour in 1 cup of water and then add the eggs. Make sure to lock the lid and set the time for 10 minutes at high pressure.

Release the pressure as you want and then separate the egg from the water to cool. Peel and cut in half.

Nutrition:

Calories – 60

Protein – 6 g.

Fat – 4 g.

Carbs – 0 g.

Banana French Toast

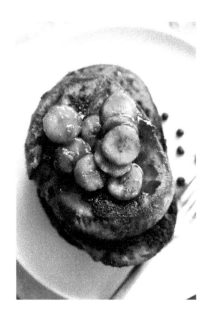

Preparation Time: 5 minutes

Cooking Time: 20 minutes

Servings: 4

Ingredients:

Butter1 tbsp.

Steel cut oats1 cup

Water3 cups

Salt to taste

Raisins¾ cup

Directions:

Turn on to sauté function and add the butter.

When it is melted, add the toast and the oats. Stir and make it dark.

Now add the water and salt. Stir and close the lid. Manually set the time for 10 minutes.

When it is done, take off the lid and stir with raisins. Sit for 5 to 10 minutes to allow the oats thicken.

Serve with your favorite topping.

Nutrition:

Calories – 180

Protein – 5 g.

Fat – 5 g.

Carbs – 31 g.

Delicious Scotch Eggs

Preparation Time: 5 minutes

Cooking Time: 30 minutes

Servings: 4

Ingredients:

Egg4

Ground sausage1lb.

Vegetable oil1 tbsp.

Directions:

Take your instant pot and add the rack that came with it. Pour in 1 cup of water and then place the eggs.

Make sure to lock the lid and set the time for 10 minutes at high pressure.

Release the pressure as you want and then separate the eggs from the water to cool. Peel and wrap the eggs with the sausages around the eggs. Remove the rack and Put the instant potto sauté function and sauté the eggs in the vegetable oil. Set aside.

Set the rack back in the instant pot and add the water. Now place the eggs and set the time for 6 minutes.

Yap, ready

Nutrition:

Calories – 288

Protein – 27 g.

Fat – 16 g.

Carbs – 1 g.

Delicious Yogurt with Fruit

Preparation Time: 5 minutes

Cooking Time: 45 minutes

Servings: 6

Ingredients:

Milk1 gallon

Greek yogurt½ cup

Vanilla bean paste2 tbsp.

Fruit2 cups

Sugar1 cup

Directions:

Transfer the milk in your instant pot and press the yogurt button. Set the time for 45 minutes.

Turn off the cooker and when it reaches 115 F, add the yogurt and the vanilla bean paste.

Switch on the instant pot and set the yogurt button again. Allow to cook for 8 hours.

Transfer the yogurt into convenient sized jar and place in the refrigerator. Leave it for 1-day.

When you are about to serve, boil the fruit with the sugar and cool before serving.

Place the yogurt in the serving cup and place the fruit on the top of the yogurt.

Nutrition:

Calories – 232

Protein – 10 g.

Fat – 0.5 g.

Carbs – 34 g.

Breakfast Quinoa

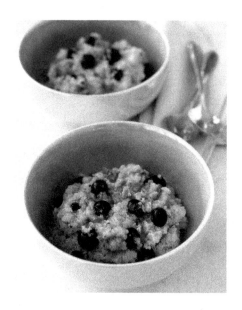

Preparation Time: 5 minutes

Cooking Time: 30 minutes

Servings: 6

Ingredients:

Quinoa1 ½ cups

Water2 ¼ cups

Maple syrup2 tbsp.

Vanilla½ tbsp.

Cinnamon¼ tsp.

Salt to taste

Directions:

Add all the ingredients into the instant pot and close the lid. Manually set the time to 1 minute at high pressure. Allow to cook.

Turn off the cooker and naturally release the pressure.

Fluff and serve with berries, milk and sliced almonds.

Nutrition:

Calories – 400

Protein – 7 g.

Fat – 2 g.

Carbs – 22 g.

Easy Buckwheat Porridge

Preparation Time: 5 minutes

Cooking Time: 30 minutes

Servings: 4

Ingredients:

Raw buckwheat groats1 cup

Rice milk3 cups

Banana1, sliced

Raisins¼ cup

Ground cinnamon1 tsp.

Vanilla½ tsp.

Directions:

Place the buckwheat, cinnamon, vanilla, raisins, banana and rice milk into the instant pot.

Make sure to lock the lid and set the time for 6 minutes at high pressure.

When the cooking is done, allow naturally release the pressure and then stir the porridge.

When it is time to serve, add more rice milk to get the desire consistency.

Nutrition:

Calories – 300

Protein – 7 g.

Fat – 14 g.

Carbs – 34 g.

Almond Steel-Cut Oatmeal

Preparation Time: 5 minutes

Cooking Time: 20 minutes

Servings: 2

Ingredients:

1 tsp olive oil

1 cup steel-cut oats

1½ cups water

¾ cup almond milk

Directions:

Warm oil on Sauté, until foaming. Add oats and cook as you stir until soft and toasted. Press Cancel. Add milk, salt and water and stir.
Seal the lid, and Press Porridge. Cook for 12 minutes on High Pressure. Fix steam vent to Venting to release pressure quickly. Open the lid. Add oats as you stir to mix any extra liquid.

Nutrition:

Calories – 350

Protein – 14 g.

Fat – 8 g., Carbs – 26 g.

Breakfast Mix

Preparation Time: 5 minutes

Cooking Time: 15 minutes

Servings: 2

Ingredients:

2 bacon slices, chopped

3 ham slices, chopped

½ cup chicken broth

1 cup frozen peas

1 tsp garlic powder

1 tsp onion powder

Salt and black pepper to taste

1 tbsp chopped parsley

Directions:

Fix your Instant Pot to Sauté mode and adjust to medium heat. Put in the bacon and cook until crispy, 5 minutes. Mix in ham and heat through, 1 minute. Top with chicken broth, frozen peas, garlic powder, onion powder, salt, and black pepper.

Seal the lid, select Manual/Pressure Cook mode on High, and set cooking time to 1 minute. After cooking, do a quick pressure release to let out steam, and unlock the lid. Dish food, garnish with parsley and serve warm.

Nutrition:

Calories – 450

Protein – 29 g.

Fat – 18 g.

Carbs – 21 g.

Maple Pumpkin Steel-Cut Oatmeal

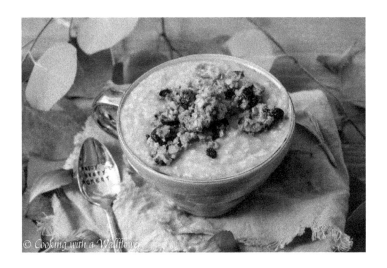

© Cooking with a Wallflower

Preparation Time: 5 minutes
Cooking Time: 25 minutes

Servings: 2

Ingredients:

1 tbsp butter

2 cups steel cut oats

¼ tsp cinnamon

3 cups water

1 cup pumpkin puree

½ tsp salt

3 tbsp maple syrup

½cup pumpkin seeds, toasted

Directions:

Melt butter on Sauté. Add in cinnamon, oats, salt, pumpkin puree and water.

Seal the lid, select Porridge and cook for 10 minutes on High Pressure to get a few bite oats or for 14 minutes to form oats that are soft. Do a quick release. Open the lid and stir in maple syrup. Top with pumpkin seeds to serve.

Nutrition:

Calories – 375

Protein – 22 g.

Fat – 14 g.

Carbs – 27 g.

Coffee Steel-Cut Oatmeal

Preparation Time: 5 minutes

Cooking Time: 20 minutes

Servings: 2-4

Ingredients:

3 ½ cups milk

½ cup raw peanuts

1 cup steel-cut oats

¼ cup agave syrup

1 tsp coffee

1 ½ tsp ground ginger

1 ¼ tsp ground cinnamon

½ tsp salt

¼ tsp ground allspice

¼ tsp ground cardamom

1 tsp vanilla extract

Directions:

With a blender, puree peanuts and milk to obtain a smooth consistency. Transfer into the cooker. To the peanuts mixture, add in agave syrup, oats, ginger, allspice, cinnamon, salt, cardamom, tea leaves, and cloves, and mix well.

Make sure to close the lid and cook on High Pressure for 12 minutes. Let pressure to release naturally on completing the cooking cycle. Add vanilla extract to the oatmeal and stir well before serving.

Nutrition:

Calories – 350

Protein – 26 g.

Fat – 17 g.

Carbs – 19 g.

Vanilla Carrot Cake Oatmeal

Preparation Time: 5 minutes

Cooking Time: 20 minutes

Servings: 2

Ingredients:

2 cups milk

1 cup old fashioned rolled oats

1 cup shredded carrots + extra for garnishing

2 tbsp maple syrup

1 tsp cinnamon

¼ tsp ground ginger

1/8 tsp grated nutmeg

1 tsp vanilla extract

¼ cup chopped dates

¼ cup chopped pecans

Directions:

Pour milk, oats, carrots, maple syrup, cinnamon, ginger, nutmeg, and vanilla into inner pot. Seal the lid, select Manualon High, and set cooking time to 3 minutes.

After cooking, perform natural pressure release for 10 minutes, then a quick pressure release to let out the remaining steam. Unlock lid, stir in dates and pecans, and spoon oatmeal into bowls. Garnish with remaining carrots and serve.

Nutrition:

Calories – 425

Protein – 31 g.

Fat – 22 g.

Carbs – 27 g.

Coconut Porridge

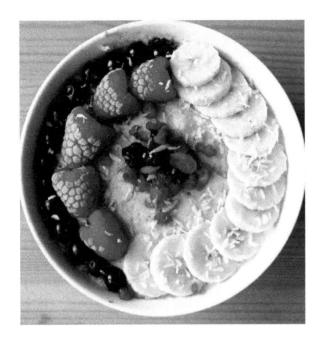

Preparation Time: 5 minutes

Cooking Time: 20 minutes

Servings: 2

Ingredients:

1 cup rye flakes

A pinch of salt

1 ¼ cups coconut milk

1 tsp vanilla extract

2 tbsp maple syrup

¾ cup frozen black currants

Directions:

In inner pot, combine rye flakes, salt, coconut milk, water, vanilla, and maple syrup. Seal the lid, select Manual/Pressure Cook on High, and set time to 5 minutes. After cooking, perform natural pressure release for 10 minutes. Stir and spoon porridge into serving bowls. Top with black currants and serve warm.

Nutrition:

Calories – 340

Protein – 24 g.

Fat – 16 g.

Carbs – 19 g.

Easy Beef Sandwiches

Preparation Time: 10 minutes

Cooking Time: 50 minutes

Servings: 2

Ingredients:

½ pound beef roast

½ tbsp olive oil

¼ onion, chopped

1 garlic clove, minced

2 tbsp dry red wine

½ cup beef broth stock

¼ tsp dried oregano

4 slices Fontina cheese

2 split hoagie rolls

Directions:

Season the beef with salt and pepper. Warm oil on Sauté and brown the beef for 2 to 3 minutes per side. Set aside on a plate. Add in the onion and cook for 3 minutes, until translucent. Stir in garlic and cook for one minute until soft.

Add red wine to deglaze. Scrape the cooking surface to remove any brown sections of the food using a wooden spoon's flat edge. Mix in beef broth and take back the juices and beef to your cooker.

Over the meat, scatter some oregano. Make sure to cover the lid and cook on High Pressure for 30 minutes.

Naturally release the pressure for 10 minutes. Preheat a broiler. Take the beef to a cutting board and slice. Roll the beef and top with onions. Each sandwich should be topped with 2 slices fontina cheese.

Place the sandwiches under the broiler for a couple of minutes until the cheese melts.

Nutrition:

Calories – 700

Protein – 55 g.

Fat – 42 g.

Carbs – 49 g.

Raspberry Yogurt

Preparation Time: 5 minutes

Cooking Time: 30 minutes

Servings: 6-8

Ingredients:

1 pound hulled and halved raspberries

1 cup sugar

3 tbsp gelatin

1 tbsp fresh orange juice

8 cups milk

¼ cup Greek yogurt containing active cultures

Directions:

In a bowl, mash raspberries with a potato masher. Add sugar and stir well to dissolve; let soak for 30 minutes at room temperature. Add in orange juice and gelatin and mix well until dissolved.

Remove the mixture and place in a sealable container, close, and allow to sit for 12 to 24 hours at room temperature before placing in a refrigerator. Refrigerate for a maximum of 2 weeks.

Into the cooker, add milk and close the lid. The steam vent should be set to Venting then to Sealing.

Select Yogurt until "Boil" is displayed on the readings. When complete there will be a display of "Yogurt" on the screen. Open the lid and using a food thermometer ensure the milk temperature is at least 185°F.

Transfer the steel pot to a wire rack and allow cool for 30 minutes until milk has reached 110°F.

In a bowl, mix ½ cup warm milk and yogurt. Transfer the mixture into the remaining warm milk and stir without having to scrape the steel pot's bottom.

Take the pot back to the base of the pot and seal the lid. Select Yogurt mode and cook for 8 hours. Allow the yogurt to chill in a refrigerator for 1-2 hours. Transfer the chilled yogurt to a large bowl and Stir in fresh raspberry jam.

Nutrition:

Calories – 320, Protein – 25 g., Fat – 8 g., Carbs – 14 g.

Chickpea & Avocado Burritos

Preparation Time: 5 minutes

Cooking Time: 30 minutes

Servings: 2

Ingredients:

1 tbsp coconut oil

1 medium red onion, finely chopped

1 red bell pepper, deseeded and chopped

1 garlic clove, minced

1 tsp cumin powder

1 ½ cups canned chickpeas, drained

½ cup vegetable broth

Salt and black pepper to taste

3 corn tortillas

1 large avocado, halved, pitted, and chopped

½ cup shredded red cabbage

3 tbsp chopped cilantro

3 tbsp tomato salsa

½ cup sour cream

Directions:

Put the instant potto Sauté and adjust to medium heat. Heat coconut oil in inner pot and sauté onion and bell pepper until softened, 4 minutes. Add garlic, cumin, and cook for 1 minute or until fragrant.

Mix in chickpeas, heat through for 1 minute with frequent stirring, and pour in vegetable broth. Season with salt and black pepper. Seal the lid, select Manual/Pressure Cook on High, and set cooking time to 8 minutes.

After cooking, perform natural pressure release for 10 minutes, then a quick pressure release to let out the remaining steam. Unlock the lid, stir, and adjust taste with salt and black pepper. Turn Instant Pot off. Place tortillas on a flat surface and divide chickpea filling at the center. Top with avocados, cabbage, cilantro, salsa, and sour cream. Wrap, tuck ends, and slice in halves. Serve for lunch.

Nutrition:

Calories – 650, Protein – 49 g.Fat – 32 g.
Carbs – 44 g.

Easy Oatmeal Bowls with Raspberries

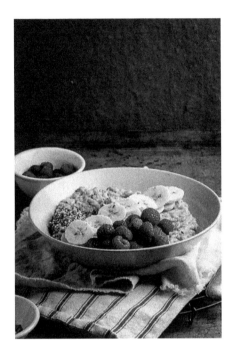

Preparation Time: 5 minutes

Cooking Time: 20 minutes

Servings: 2

Ingredients:

1 cup steel-cut oats

1 ½ cups milk

2 tbsp honey

½ tsp vanilla extract

A pinch salt

Fresh raspberries, for topping

Toasted Brazil nuts, for topping

Directions:

Add the oats, milk, honey, vanilla, and salt into inner pot. Seal the lid, select Manual/Pressure Cook mode, and set cooking time to 6 minutes on High. When done, perform a quick pressure release to let out the steam. Unlock the lid and stir the oatmeal. Divide between serving bowls and top with raspberries and toasted Brazil nuts to serve.

Nutrition:

Calories – 250

Protein – 18 g.

Fat – 8 g.

Carbs – 16 g.

Super-Fast Pomegranate Porridge

Preparation Time: 5 minutes

Cooking Time: 5 minutes

Servings: 2

Ingredients:

1 cup oats

1 cup pomegranate juice

1 cup water

1 tbsp. pomegranate molasses

Sea salt to taste

Directions:

Place the water, oats, salt, and juice in your Instant Pot. Stir to combine and seal the lid. Select Porridge, and cook for 3 minutes on High pressure. Once ready, do a quick pressure release. Cautiously open the lid and stir in the pomegranate molasses. Serve immediately.

Nutrition:

Calories – 175

Protein – 14 g.

Fat – 6 g.,Carbs – 11 g.

Chicken Sandwiches with BBQ Sauce

Preparation Time: 10 minutes

Cooking Time: 45 minutes

Servings: 2-4

Ingredients:

4 chicken thighs, boneless and skinless

Salt to taste

2 cups barbecue sauce

1 onion, minced

2 garlic cloves, minced

2 tbsp minced fresh parsley

1 tbsp lemon juice

1 tbsp mayonnaise

1½ cups iceberg lettuce, shredded

4 burger buns

Directions:

Season the chicken with salt, and transfer into the pot. Add in garlic, onion and barbeque sauce. Coat the chicken by turning in the sauce. Make sure to cover the lid and cook on High Pressure for 15 minutes.

Do a natural release for 10 minutes. Use two forks to strip the chicken and mix into the sauce. Press Keep Warm and let the mixture to simmer for 15 minutes to thicken the sauce, until desired consistency.

In a bowl, mix lemon juice, mayonnaise, salt, and parsley; toss lettuce into the mixture to coat. Separate the chicken in equal parts to match the sandwich buns; apply lettuce for topping and complete the sandwiches.

Nutrition:

Calories – 750

Protein – 63 g.

Fat – 49 g.

Carbs – 57 g.

Squash Tart Oatmeal

Preparation Time: 5 minutes

Cooking Time: 35 minutes

Servings: 2-4

Ingredients:

3 ½ cups coconut milk

1 cup steel-cut oats

1 cup shredded butternut squash

½ cup sultanas

⅓ cup honey

1 tsp ground cinnamon

¾ tsp ground ginger

½ tsp salt

½ tsp orange zest

¼ tsp ground nutmeg

¼ cup toasted walnuts, chopped

½ tsp vanilla extract

Directions:

In the cooker, mix sultanas, orange zest, ginger, milk, honey, squash, salt, oats, and nutmeg. Make sure to cover the lid and cook on High Pressure for 12 minutes. Do a natural release for 10 minutes. Into the oatmeal, stir in the vanilla extract and sugar. Top with walnuts and serve.

Nutrition:

Calories – 310

Protein – 25 g.

Fat – 16 g.

Carbs – 21 g.

Cherry Oatmeal

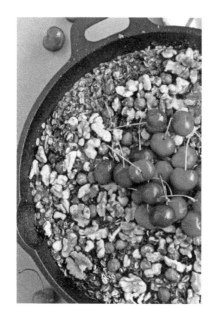

Preparation Time: 5 minutes

Cooking Time: 20 minutes

Servings: 2

Ingredients:

2 cups milk

1 cup old fashioned rolled oats

1 tbsp cocoa powder

3 tbsp maple syrup

½ cup dried cherries

Greek Yogurt for topping

¼ cup chopped walnuts

Directions: Pour milk, oats, cocoa powder, maple syrup, and cherries into inner pot. Seal the lid, select Manual/Pressure Cook on High, and set cooking time to 3 minutes. After cooking, perform natural pressure release for 10 minutes, then a quick pressure release to let out the remaining steam. Unlock the lid, stir, and spoon oatmeal into serving bowls. Top with Greek yogurt, walnuts, and serve warm.

Nutrition:

Calories – 330

Protein – 26 g.

Fat – 18 g.

Carbs – 21 g.

Mushroom & Cheese Oatmeal

Preparation Time: 5 minutes

Cooking Time: 35 minutes

Servings: 2

Ingredients:

1 tbsp butter

1 cup sliced cremini mushrooms

1 garlic clove, minced

1 tsp thyme leaves

Salt and black pepper to taste

1 cup chopped baby kale

1 cup old fashioned rolled oats

2 cups vegetable broth

¼ tsp red pepper flakes

¼ cup crumbled feta cheese

Directions:

Put the instant potto Sauté and adjust to medium heat. Melt butter in inner pot and sauté mushrooms until slightly softened, 4 to 5 minutes. Stir in garlic, thyme, salt, and black pepper. Cook until fragrant, 3 minutes.

Mix in kale to wilt; stir in oats, vegetable broth, and red pepper flakes. Seal the lid, select Manual/Pressure Cook on High, and set cooking time to 3 minutes.

After cooking, perform natural pressure release for 10 minutes. Unlock the lid, stir, and adjust taste with salt and black pepper. Dish oatmeal into serving bowls and top with feta cheese. Serve warm.

Nutrition:

Calories – 320

Protein – 25 g.

Fat – 17 g.

Carbs – 22 g.

Egg Croissants

Preparation Time: 5 minutes

Cooking Time: 8 minutes

Servings: 2

Ingredients:

4 large eggs

Salt and pepper to taste

4 slices of bacon,cut into small pieces

5 tablespoons shredded cheddar cheese

1 green scallion, diced

4 croissants

Directions:

Place a steamer basket inside the instant pot and pour in 1½ cups water.

Whip the eggs in a bowl. Add the bacon pieces, cheese, and scallion to the eggs. Mix well.

Divided the mixture into 4 muffin cups. Transfer the filled muffin cups onto the steamer basket. Shut the lid and cook at high pressure for 8 minutes.

When the cooking is complete, do a natural pressure release for 5 minutes. Quick-release the remaining pressure.

Lift the muffin cups out the instant pot.

Slice 4 croissants in half and stuff with the muffin cup content.

Nutrition:

Calories – 482

Protein – 21 g.

Fat – 29.9 g.

Carbs – 31.5 g.

Broccoli Egg Morning

Preparation Time: 5-8 minutes

Cooking Time: 8 minutes

Servings: 2

Ingredients:

3 eggs, whisked

½ cup broccoli florets

A pinch garlic powder

2 tablespoons tomatoes

1 clove garlic, minced

½ small yellow onion, chopped

½ red bell pepper, chopped

2 tablespoons cheese, grated

A pinch chili powder

2 tablespoons onions

2 tablespoons parsley

Pepper and salt as needed

Directions:

Take your 3-quart instant pot; open the top lid.

Plug it and turn it on.

Open the top lid; grease inside cooking surface using a cooking spray.

In a bowl, whisk the eggs.

Add remaining ingredients except for the cheese.

Season with pepper and salt.

In the cooking pot area, add the mixture.

Make sure to cover the lid and seal its valve.

Press "STEAM" setting. Set cooking time to 5 minutes.

Let the recipe to cook for the set cooking time.

After the time ends, press "CANCEL" and then press "QPR (Quick Pressure Release)".

Instant pot wills quickly releaser the pressure.

Open the lid; put the dish in serving plates. Top with the cheese.

Serve and enjoy!

Nutrition:

Calories – 376

Protein – 23 g.

Fat – 28 g.

Carbs – 39 g.

Broccoli Cheese Omelet

Preparation Time: 5 minutes

Cooking Time: 5 minutes

Servings: 2

Ingredients:

1 clove garlic, minced

½ small yellow onion, chopped

½ red bell pepper, chopped

3 eggs, whisked

½ cup broccoli florets

A pinch garlic powder

2 tablespoons tomatoes, diced

2 tablespoons onions, diced

2 tablespoons parsley

2 tablespoons cheese, grated

A pinch chili powder

Black pepper and salt, to taste

Cooking spray, as needed

Directions:

Place your instant pot on a dry surface.

Open the lid; grease inside cooking surface with cooking spray.

In a medium bowl, thoroughly whisk the eggs.

Add remaining ingredients except for the cheese.

Season with black pepper and salt.

Add the mixture to the instant pot.

Ensure to lock the lid and seal it properly.

Press STEAM; set timer to 5 minutes.

The instant pot will start building pressure; allow the mixture to cook for the set time.

After the timer reaches zero, turn venting knob from sealing to the venting position. Wait until float valve drops (1-2 minutes).

Open the lid and take the food into a plate.

Top with the cheese; slice in half and serve warm.

Nutrition:

Calories – 389

Protein – 24.3 g.

Fat – 28.7 g.

Carbs – 9.8 g.

Jar Breakfast

Preparation Time: 15 minutes

Cooking Time: 5 minutes

Servings: 2

Ingredients:

4 eggs

4 pieces bacon, cooked of your preferred breakfast meat, such as sausage

4 tablespoons peach-mango salsa, divided

6 slices sharp cheese or shredded, cheese, Divided

Tater tots

Directions:

Put 1¼ cups water in the inner pot. Put enough tater tots cover the bottom of the mason jars. Crock 2 eggs in each. Poke the yolks using a fork or tip of a long thin knife. Add your choice of meats, 2 slices cheese to cover the ingredients, and 2 tablespoons salsa. Add more tater tots and top with 1 slice cheese. Tightly cover the jars with foil. Put the jars in the IP, right in the water.

Lock the lid and close the valve. Fix the Instant Pot to manual high pressure for 5 minutes. QPR when the timer beeps. Open the lid. Carefully remove the jars. Serve.

Nutrition:

Calories – 632

Protein – 38 g.

Fat – 46 g.

Carbs – 16 g.

Vanilla Peach Oats

Preparation Time: 5 minutes

Cooking Time: 3 minutes

Servings: 2

Ingredients:

1 peach, chopped

2 cups of water

1 cups rolled oats

½ teaspoon vanilla

1 tablespoon flax meal

½ tablespoon maple syrup

Directions:

Place everything in your instant pot. Stir to combine well.

Close the lid, and turn the vents to "sealed"

Press "Pressure Cook" (manual) button, use "+" or "-"button to set the timer for 3 minutes. Use "pressure level" button to set the pressure to high.

Once the timer is up, press the "cancel" button and allow the pressure to be released naturally until the float valve drops down.

Open the lid. Serve and enjoy!

Nutrition:

Calories – 193

Protein – 6.3 g.

Fat – 3.3 g.

Carbs – 27.6 g.

Pecan Pie Oatmeal

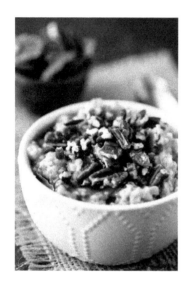

Preparation Time: 5 minutes

Cooking Time: 3 minutes

Servings: 2

Ingredients:

½ cup steel cut oats

1¾ cups water

1/8 cup half & half

2 Medjool dates, Chopped

¼ cup pecans, chopped

3 tablespoons maple syrup

½ teaspoon ground cinnamon

¼ teaspoon nutmeg

Directions:

Put all ingredients in the pot and stir.

Make sure to lock the lid and cook at high for three minutes.

When the cooking is complete, does a natural pressure release.

Serve warm with maple syrup.

Nutrition:

Calories – 230

Protein – 4 g.

Fat – 8.2 g.

Carbs – 37.1 g.

Berry Chia Oats

Preparation Time: 5 minutes

Cooking Time: 6 minutes

Servings: 2

Ingredients:

1/2 cups old fashioned oats

½ cups almond milk, unsweetened

½ cups blueberries

1 teaspoon chia seeds

Sweetener or sugar as needed

Splash of vanilla

Pinch of salt

A pinch ground cinnamon

1 ½ cups water

Directions:

In the medium bowl, thoroughly mix all the ingredients, add the bowl mixture to a pint-size jar and cover with an aluminum foil.

In the pot, slowly pour the water. Take the trivet and arrange inside it; place the jar over it.

Make sure to lock the lid and lock it. Make certain that you have sealed the valve to avoid leakage. Press "Manual" mode and put the timer for six minutes. Wait for a few minutes for the pot to build inside pressure and start cooking.

After the timer reaches zero, press "cancel" and naturally release pressure. It takes about 8-10 minutes to release pressure naturally.

Carefully open the lid and get the jar. Mix in the oatmeal; serve warm!

Nutrition:

Calories – 114

Protein – 4.5 g.

Fat – 3 g.

Carbs – 18 g.

Potato Ham Breakfast Casserole

Preparation Time: 5 minutes

Cooking Time: 16 minutes

Servings: 2

Ingredients:

1 stick butter

¼ cup milk

¼ cup sour cream

¾ pound potatoes, diced and cooked

¾ cup mixed cheese, shredded

¼ cup ham, diced

2 green onion, sliced

Black pepper and salt, as needed

Directions:

Place your instant pot on a dry surface and open the lid.

Press SAUTE; add the butter and melt it.

Mix in the onions and potato; cook; for 4 minutes until soft and translucent.

Add the milk, ham, sour cream, a pinch black pepper (ground) and salt; stir them well to coat.

Add the cheese on top.

Make sure to lock the lid and ensure it is sealed properly.

Press MANUAL; set timer to 12 minutes.

The instant pot will start building pressure; allow the mixture to cook for the set time.

After the timer reaches zero, wait for the float valve to drop. It will take 8-10 minutes.

Open the lid and put the dish into a plate.

Divide among serving plates/bowls; serve warm.

Nutrition:

Calories – 528

Protein – 13.6 g.

Fat – 27.3 g.

Carbs – 46.8 g.

Boiled Eggs

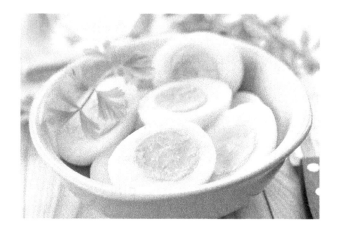

Preparation Time: 5 minutes

Cooking Time: 3-9 minutes

Servings: 2

Ingredients:

Large eggs, as much as you need

1 cup of water

Directions:

Put the IP steamer basket and pour 1 cup water in the inner pot. Put the eggs in the steamer. Close the lid and the pressure valve. Set the IP to low PRESSURE for 3-4 minutes for soft boiled, 5-7 minutes for medium-boiled, or 8-9 minutes for hard-boiled eggs.

Ready a bowl and half fill it with cold water and ice. QPR when the timer beeps. Open the lid. Transfer the eggs immediately in the ice bath. Let cool for 5 to 10 minutes .serve.

Nutrition:

Calories – 63

Protein – 5.5 g.

Fat – 4.4 g.

Carbs – 0.3 g.

Ham Sausage Quiche

Preparation Time: 5 minutes

Cooking Time: 30 minutes

Servings: 2

Ingredients:

1 cups of water

3 eggs

2 bacon slices, cooked and crumbled

¼ cup milk

1/4 cup diced ham

½ cup cooked ground sausage

½ pinch of black pepper

½ cup grated cheddar cheese

1 bunch of green onions, chopped

1 scallion, chopped

Directions:

Pour the water into your instant pot. Mix the eggs together with the salt, pepper, and milk, in a bowl. In a 1-quart baking dish, add the bacon, sausage, ham, and mix to combine.

Add the eggs in, and stir to combine again

Sprinkle with green onions and cheese.

Cover with foil and place in the instant pot.

Close the lid, and shift the vent to "sealed".

Press "pressure cook" (manual) button, use "+" or "-"button to set the timer for 30 minutes. Use "pressure level" button to set the pressure to high. Once done, press "cancel" button and turns the steam release handle to "venting" position for quick release until the float valve drops down. Open the lid. Serve warm.

Nutrition:

Calories – 396

Protein – 28.6 g.

Fat – 31.7 g.

Carbs – 4.3 g.

Conclusion

When you are on a diet trying to lose weight or manage a condition, you will be strictly confined to follow an eating plan. Such plans often place numerous demands on individuals: food may need to be boiled, other foods are forbidden, permitting you only to eat small portions and so on.

On the other hand, a lifestyle such as the Mediterranean diet is entirely stress-free. It is easy to follow because there are almost no restrictions. There is no time limit on the Mediterranean diet because it is more of a lifestyle than a diet. You do not need to stop at some point but carry on for the rest of your life. The foods that you eat under the Mediterranean model include unrefined cereals, white meats, and the occasional dairy products.

The Mediterranean lifestyle, unlike other diets, also requires you to engage with family and friends and share meals together. It has been noted that communities around the Mediterranean spend between one and two hours enjoying their meals.

This kind of bonding between family members or friends helps bring people closer together, which helps foster closer bonds hence fewer cases of depression, loneliness, or stress, all of which are precursors to chronic diseases.

You will achieve many benefits using the Instant Pot Pressure Cooker. These are just a few instances you will discover in your Mediterranean-style recipes:

Pressure cooking means that you can (on average) cook meals 75% faster than boiling/braising on the stovetop or baking and roasting in a conventional oven.

This is especially helpful for vegan meals that entail the use of dried beans, legumes, and pulses. Instead of pre-soaking these ingredients for hours before use, you can pour them directly into the Instant Pot, add water, and pressure cook these for several minutes. However, always follow your recipe carefully since they have been tested for accuracy.

Nutrients are preserved. You can use your pressure-cooking techniques using the Instant Pot to ensure the heat is evenly and quickly distributed. It is not essential to immerse the food into the water. You will provide plenty of water in the cooker for efficient steaming. You will also be saving the essential vitamins and minerals. The food won't become oxidized by the exposure of air or heat. Enjoy those fresh green veggies with their natural and vibrant colors.

The cooking elements help keep the foods fully sealed, so the steam and aromas don't linger throughout your entire home. That is a plus, especially for items such as cabbage, which throws out a distinctive smell.

You will find that beans and whole grains will have a softer texture and will have an improved taste. The meal will be cooked consistently since the Instant Pot provides even heat distribution.

You'll also save tons of time and money. You will be using much less water, and the pot is fully insulated, making it more energy-efficient when compared to boiling or steaming your foods on the stovetop. It is also less expensive than using a microwave, not to mention how much more flavorful the food will be when prepared in the Instant Pot cooker.

You can delay the cooking of your food items so you can plan ahead of time. You won't need to stand around as you await your meal. You can reduce the cooking time by reducing the 'hands-on' time. Just leave for work or a day of activities, and you will come home to a special treat. In a nutshell, the Instant Pot is:

Easy To Use

Healthy recipes for the entire family are provided.

You can make authentic one-pot recipes in your Instant Pot.

If you forget to switch on your slow cooker, you can make any meal done in a few minutes in your Instant Pot.

You can securely and smoothly cook meat from frozen.

It's a laid-back way to cook. You don't have to watch a pan on the stove or a pot in the oven.

The pressure cooking procedure develops delicious flavors swiftly.

CPSIA information can be obtained
at www.ICGtesting.com
Printed in the USA
BVHW052028120421
604747BV00005B/308